THE M

RESET DIET

COOKBOOK

Solve Menopause Challenges Deliciously and Balance Your Hormones with Recipes for a Happy and Healthy Transition

DARREN RUIZ

TABLE OF CONTENTS

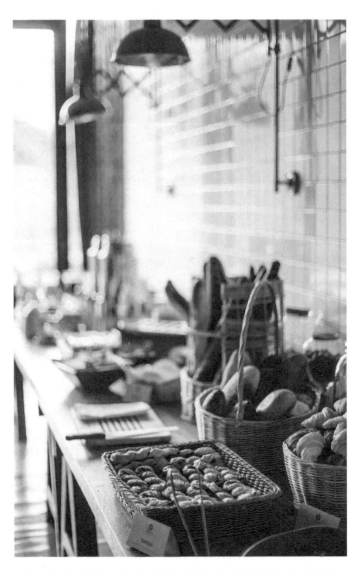

THE MENOPAUSE RESET DIET COOKBOOK

Juliet had always been the kind of woman who approached life with grace and enthusiasm. As she entered her early 40s, she expected that menopause might be on the horizon, but she never anticipated that it would arrive so soon.

The hot flashes, mood swings, and sleepless nights took her by surprise, and it felt like her body had embarked on an unexpected rollercoaster ride.

Determined to regain control of her life, Juliet turned to "The Menopause Reset Diet Cookbook." The book had been her trusted companion since the moment it arrived on her doorstep.

It offered a lifeline of information and delicious recipes tailored for menopausal women like her.

Juliet delved into the book with fervour, absorbing every word of wisdom about nutrition and wellness during menopause.

She started by adjusting her diet, focusing on hormone-balancing foods that she found in the book. She made breakfasts filled with nutrient-rich ingredients to kickstart her day with energy and vitality.

Her lunches were satisfying and nourishing, keeping her energised throughout the day. And the dinners, oh, those hormone-balancing dinners, had a soothing effect that made her evenings restful and serene.

The recipes in the book became Juliet's culinary arsenal. She prepared berry blast smoothies, chia seed pudding, and baked apples with cinnamon and walnuts.

Her friends and family marvelled at the delicious meals she served, not realising that these dishes were carefully chosen to support her menopausal journey.

As the weeks passed, Juliet noticed a transformation.

The hot flashes became less frequent, her mood swings levelled out, and she enjoyed restful nights of sleep.

She felt a renewed sense of control over her body and her life. The menopausal rollercoaster was slowing down, and she was regaining her equilibrium.

Juliet's story is a testament to the power of embracing the right diet during menopause. By adopting the principles of "The Menopause Reset Diet Cookbook," she didn't just manage her symptoms; she thrived during this life transition.

The book had become her trusted companion on the journey to health, happiness, and empowerment.

With every delicious meal she prepared, Juliet celebrated her strength, resilience, and boundless optimism. Menopause had arrived early, but it was no match for Juliet's determination to live her best life.

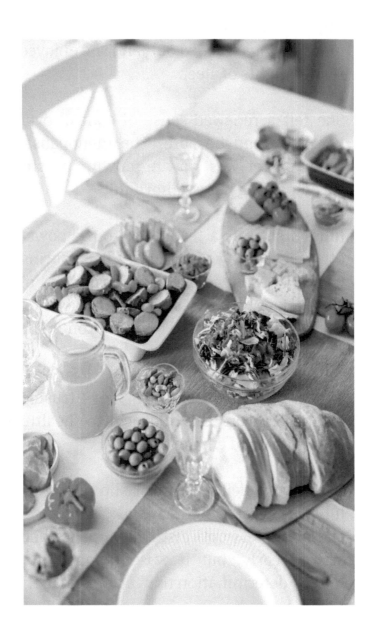

INTRODUCTION

Menopause is a transformative phase in a woman's life, a journey marked by profound physical and emotional changes. As a natural biological process, it signifies the end of a woman's reproductive years, typically occurring in her late 40s to early 50s.

Menopause is often accompanied by a range of symptoms, from hot flashes and mood swings to sleep disturbances and changes in metabolism. While it is a universal experience for women, its effects can be highly individual, making it a unique and often challenging journey.

This introduction sets the stage for our exploration of menopause and how nutrition plays a pivotal role in helping women navigate this significant life transition.

We will delve into the physical and emotional aspects of menopause, the changes it brings, and how a well-considered diet can be a powerful tool in managing and even thriving during this transformative phase.

Understanding Menopause

Menopause, from the Greek words "menos" (month) and "pausis" (to stop), is defined as the permanent cessation of menstruation.

It marks the end of a woman's reproductive capacity and the closing of one chapter in her life while opening another.

This natural transition is driven by a decrease in the production of key hormones, primarily oestrogen and progesterone, which regulate the menstrual cycle.

The symptoms of menopause can vary widely among women, and their severity can range from mildly inconvenient to significantly disruptive. The most common symptoms include:

Hot Flashes: Sudden sensations of heat that may cause redness, sweating, and discomfort.

Night Sweats: Hot flashes that occur during sleep, often leading to sleep disturbances.

Mood Swings: Hormonal fluctuations can lead to mood swings, irritability, and even depression.

Vaginal Dryness: A decrease in oestrogen can result in vaginal dryness, leading to discomfort during intercourse.

Sleep Disturbances: Insomnia and disrupted sleep patterns can be a significant challenge.

Changes in Metabolism: Many women experience weight gain and changes in body composition.

Bone Health: A decrease in oestrogen can lead to a decrease in bone density, potentially increasing the risk of osteoporosis.

Understanding these symptoms and their underlying causes is the first step in effectively managing menopause.

It's essential for women to recognize that they are not alone in this journey, and there are ways to address these challenges with confidence and grace.

The Power of Nutrition in Menopause

Nutrition is a fundamental aspect of overall health and well-being, and it becomes even more critical during menopause.

A well-balanced and thoughtfully planned diet can help women manage the physical and emotional changes that accompany this life phase.

Hormone Balance: Nutrition plays a vital role in hormone balance. Certain foods, such as those rich in phytoestrogens (plant compounds similar to oestrogen), can help stabilise hormone levels.

Additionally, a diet that supports healthy insulin and blood sugar levels can assist in managing metabolic changes.

Bone Health: Maintaining strong and healthy bones is essential, especially as oestrogen levels decline. A diet rich in calcium and vitamin D can help support bone health and reduce the risk of osteoporosis.

Heart Health: Menopausal women are at an increased risk of heart disease. A heart-healthy diet can help manage cholesterol levels and reduce this risk.

Weight Management: As metabolism changes, many women face weight-related challenges during menopause. A nutritionally balanced diet can support healthy weight management.

Mood and Emotional Well-being: Nutrition can also have a profound impact on mood and emotional well-being. Certain nutrients and dietary patterns can help alleviate mood swings and improve mental health.

Throughout this book, we will explore the specific nutrients, foods, and dietary strategies that can make a positive difference during menopause.

We'll provide you with a wide range of recipes designed to address common menopausal symptoms, from meals that can help manage hot flashes to those that support bone health and mood stabilisation.

CHAPTER 1

Menopause Unveiled

In this vital chapter, we begin the trip of unveiling the mystifications of menopause, a natural and significant life transition for women.

Menopause is a phase that every woman will face, marking the end of her reproductive times, but its instantiations are far from universal, as symptoms can vary extensively.

We'll claw into the different array of symptoms and the profound impact they can have on women's lives.

Also, we will explore the common causes of menopause, slipping light on the natural processes that bolster this metamorphosis.

Menopause Symptoms and Their Impact

Menopause is much further than the conclusion of period; it's a profound and complex process that triggers a series of hormonal, physical, and emotional changes.

Understanding these symptoms and their implicit impact on a woman's life is essential for effectively navigating this life transition.

Hot Flashes: The Fiery interferers

Hot flashes are one of the most extensively honoured and generally educated symptoms of menopause. They manifest as unforeseen sensations of heat, frequently accompanied by sweating and flushing.

These" fiery interferers" can disrupt diurnal life, causing discomfort and embarrassment.

The underpinning hormonal oscillations, specifically the drop in oestrogen, spark these occurrences.

Night Sweats: Sleep Disturbance and Discomfort

Hot flashes do not just strike during the day; they can foray a woman's nights as well. Night sweats are basically hot flashes that occur during sleep, leading to intruded and disintegrated sleep patterns. This sleep disturbance can have a cascading impact on energy situations, mood, and overall well- being.

Mood Swings: The Emotional Rollercoaster

The hormonal oscillations associated with menopause can give rise to mood swings and emotional turbulence. Women may witness heightened perversity, mood swings, and indeed bouts of depression.

The emotional rollercoaster can be one of the most gruelling aspects of menopause, affecting not only the individual but also those around her.

Vaginal Blankness: Closeness and Comfort

A drop in oestrogen situations during menopause can lead to vaginal blankness. This can affect discomfort during intercourse and impact closeness and sexual satisfaction.

Understanding and addressing this symptom is pivotal for maintaining a healthy sexual relationship.

Sleep Disturbances: The Insomnia Challenge

Menopausal women frequently struggle with wakefulness and disintegrated sleep patterns.

The interplay of hormonal changes, night sweats, and mood swings can make falling and staying asleep a daunting challenge. A peaceful night's sleep is essential for overall well- being, and these sleep disturbances can affect a woman's energy and cognitive function during the day.

Changes in Metabolism: Battling the Waistline

Metabolic changes are a common circumstance during menopause. numerous women witness weight gain, particularly around the waist.

This change in body composition is frequently pertained to as the" menopausal middle," and it can be both frustrating and gruelling to manage.

Bone Health: Guarding Against Osteoporosis

As oestrogen situations decline, so does bone viscosity.

Maintaining strong and healthy bones is pivotal for precluding osteoporosis, a condition characterised by brittle bones that are prone to fractures.

Understanding the relationship between menopause and bone health is vital for women's long- term well- being. Understanding the diversity and implicit inflexibility of these symptoms is the first step in managing menopause effectively.

It's important to fete that every woman's menopause experience is unique. Some may sail through with minimum dislocations, while others may find themselves facing a myriad of challenges.

Knowledge is the key to commission, and through understanding these symptoms, women can take visionary way to address them and recapture control over their lives.

Common Causes of Menopause

Menopause is a natural and ineluctable part of a woman's life cycle, but understanding its causes provides precious perceptivity into this metamorphosis.

While the root cause of menopause is natural and linked to hormonal changes, there are several common pathways through which menopause occurs.

Natural Menopause: The Biological timepiece

The most common cause of menopause is natural menopause, which occurs as a result of the natural timepiece.

As women age, their ovaries produce smaller hormones, leading to the end of period and the onset of menopause.

Surgical Menopause: The Intervention

In some cases, menopause may be touched off by surgical intervention, similar as a hysterectomy, where the ovaries are removed.

Surgical menopause is frequently abrupt and can result in further violent symptoms due to the unforeseen drop in hormone situations.

Chemotherapy and Radiation: Induced Menopause

Cancer treatments like chemotherapy and radiation can damage the ovaries, leading to early menopause.

This can happen at any age, and the symptoms can be particularly challenging for women dealing with a cancer opinion.

Unseasonable Menopause: Early appearance

Unseasonable menopause is a condition where menopause occurs before the age of 40. It can be the result of inheritable factors, autoimmune conditions, or certain medical treatments.

Understanding the causes of menopause sheds light on the unique gests of women going through this transition.

It's essential for women to grasp the complications of their menopause trip, as this knowledge can empower them to take charge of their health and well- being.

In the posterior chapters of this book, we will claw into the part of nutrition in managing these symptoms and icing a smooth and balanced transition through menopause.

We'll give a wealth of knowledge, expert advice, and a variety of succulent fashions acclimatised to address the unique challenges of this phase in a woman's life.

Our thing is to equip women with the tools they need to embrace menopause as an occasion for growth, health, and a renewed sense of well- being.

CHAPTER 2

The Menopause Reset result

In this vital chapter, we explore" The Menopause Reset Solution," a holistic and multi-faceted approach to navigating the intricate trip of menopause.

Menopause is a transformative phase that touches every aspect of a woman's life, from physical changes to emotional oscillations.

Understanding that a one- size- fits- all approach does not work, we claw into how a holistic perspective can empower women to embrace this life transition with grace and confidence.

Also, we will uncover the critical part of nutrition in restoring hormonal balance and icing a smooth trip through menopause.

A Holistic Approach to Menopause

Menopause isn't simply a medical condition; it's a profound life transition that encompasses physical, emotional, and cerebral changes.

A holistic approach recognizes the complexity of this phase and takes into account the interconnectedness of these rudiments.

Physical Well- being: Embracing Change

Physical well- being during menopause is multifaceted. It includes addressing symptoms similar as hot flashes, night sweats, and changes in metabolism. A holistic approach involves a comprehensive evaluation of physical health, including bone health, cardiovascular health, and maintaining a healthy weight.

It's essential to nurture the body during this phase, understanding that it's witnessing significant change.

Emotional Wellness: Nurturing the Mind and Heart

Emotional hardiness is a pivotal element of menopause. Mood swings, perversity, and indeed depression can impact a woman's emotional state.

A holistic approach to menopause involves strategies to promote emotional well- being, similar as awareness, stress reduction, and embracing positive psychology.

Cerebral commission: A New morning

Menopause represents a profound transition, a moment of stepping into a new phase of life.

A holistic approach recognizes this cerebral aspect and encourages women to see it as a time of commission, growth, and tone- discovery.

It's a period of reassessment and reconsidering precedences and pretensions.

Hormonal Balance: The cornerstone of Menopause Management

Hormonal oscillations are at the heart of menopause. Oestrogen, progesterone, and other hormones play a vital part in the symptoms endured during this phase.

A holistic approach recognizes that hormonal balance is the cornerstone to menopause operation.

It seeks to address these imbalances through a combination of life, nutrition, and, in some cases, medical interventions.

The part of Nutrition in Hormone Balance

Nutrition is an important and frequently underutilised tool in managing hormonal balance during menopause. Understanding the part of nutrition in hormone balance is abecedarian to The Menopause Reset Solution.

Phytoestrogens: Plant Abettors in Hormone Balance

Phytoestrogens are factory composites that mimic the goods of oestrogen in the body. They can help stabilise hormonal oscillations during menopause. Foods rich in phytoestrogens include soy products, flaxseeds, and legumes.

Nutrient-thick Foods: Fueling Hormone Health

A diet rich in nutrient- thick foods can support hormone health during menopause.

This includes a cornucopia of fruits, vegetables, whole grains, and spare proteins. These foods give essential vitamins and minerals that play a part in hormonal balance.

Omega- 3 Adipose Acids: The Hormone-Healthy Fats

Omega- 3 adipose acids, set up in adipose fish, flaxseeds, and walnuts, have anti-inflammatory parcels that can help palliate some menopausal symptoms, similar as common pain and mood swings.

Antioxidants: Defense Against Oxidative Stress

Antioxidants cover the body from oxidative stress, which can complicate menopausal symptoms. Berries, dark leafy flora, and other antioxidant-rich foods should be a part of the menopausal diet.

Aware Eating: A Path to Emotional Balance

Aware eating isn't just about what you eat but how you eat. It encourages present-moment mindfulness and fosters a healthy relationship with food. This approach can reduce stress and emotional eating, promoting emotional balance during menopause.

Strategies for nutritive Hormone Balance

In The Menopause Reset Solution, we will present a variety of strategies and practical tips for achieving nutritive hormone balance during menopause.

These strategies will encompass mess planning, portion control, and incorporating menopause-friendly foods into your diurnal diet.

Hormone- Balancing fashions: Delicious and nutritional

We'll give a wide array of hormone-balancing fashions designed to address the common symptoms of menopause. These fashions won't only support hormonal balance but also offer scrumptious and satisfying options for breakfast, lunch, regale, and snacks.

Mess Plans: Guiding Your trip

Mess plans acclimatised to menopausal women will be an integral part of this chapter. These plans will give a clear roadmap for achieving nutritive hormone balance throughout the week.

Grocery Shopping Tips: opting Menopause-Friendly Foods

Navigating the grocery store can be inviting, but we will offer guidance on opting the right foods to support hormonal balance.

This includes choosing fresh yield, spare proteins, and whole grains.

Aware Eating Ways: Nurturing Emotional Balance

Emotional well- being during menopause is frequently overlooked but vital for a positive experience. aware eating ways will be introduced to help women manage stress and emotional eating during this phase.

The Menopause Reset Solution is designed to give a comprehensive approach to menopause that recognizes the complexity of this life transition.

We understand that every woman's experience is unique, and our holistic approach seeks to empower women with the knowledge and tools demanded to thrive during menopause.

By embracing this holistic perspective and understanding the part of nutrition in hormone balance, women can navigate menopause with grace, adaptability, and an advanced sense of overall well- being.

In the following chapters, we will claw deeper into nutrition, offering practical fashions, mess plans, and guidance to help women take charge of their menopause trip and rediscover the power of a balanced and nutritional diet.

CHAPTER 3

<u>Breakfasts for Hormonal Harmony</u>

Breakfast, often referred to as "the most important meal of the day," plays a crucial role in maintaining hormonal balance and overall well-being during menopause.

A nourishing breakfast sets the tone for the day, providing essential nutrients, energy, and emotional stability. In this chapter, we will explore morning nutritional strategies that focus on hormone balance and emotional well-being.

We'll delve into ten hormone-balancing breakfast recipes, complete with ingredients, preparation methods, nutritional value, and cooking times. Each recipe is carefully crafted to provide the nutrients necessary for a harmonious start to the day.

Hormonal Harmony through Nutrition

As hormone fluctuations are a central aspect of menopause, it's vital to prioritise foods that can help regulate these changes.

Hormonal balance can alleviate some of the most common menopausal symptoms and contribute to emotional well-being.

A balanced breakfast can:

Stabilise blood sugar levels, reducing mood swings and irritability.

Provide essential vitamins and minerals to support overall health.

Supply the body with necessary energy for daily activities.

Alleviate hot flashes and night sweats by promoting hormone stability.

By focusing on nutrient-dense and hormone-balancing foods, your breakfast can become a powerful tool for hormonal harmony during menopause.

Hormone-Balancing Breakfast Recipes

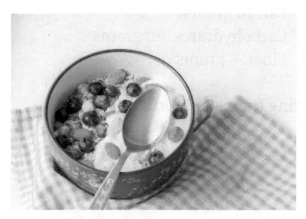

Greek Yogurt Bowl

Ingredients:
- 1 cup Greek yogurt
- 1/4 cup berries
- 1/4 cup nuts or seeds
- 1 tablespoon ground flaxseed
- 1 teaspoon honey or maple syrup (optional)

Preparation:
- Combine all ingredients in a bowl and mix well.Enjoy!

Nutritional value (per serving):
- Calories: 250
- Protein: 20 grams
- Fat: 10 grams
- Carbohydrates: 20 grams
- Fiber: 5 grams

Cooking time: 5 minutes

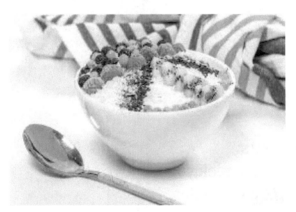

Oatmeal with Chia Seeds and Berries

Ingredients:
- 1/2 cup rolled oats
- 1 cup water or milk
- 1 tablespoon chia seeds
- 1/4 cup berries
- 1 teaspoon nuts or seeds (optional)

Preparation:
- Bring the oats and water or milk to a boil in a small saucepan.
- Reduce heat to low and simmer for 5 minutes, or until the oats are cooked through.
- Stir in the chia seeds and berries.
- Let sit for 5 minutes, or until the chia seeds have softened.
- Top with nuts or seeds (optional).Enjoy!

Nutritional value (per serving):
- Calories: 200
- Protein: 6 grams
- Fat: 5 grams
- Carbohydrates: 35 grams
- Fibre: 5 grams

Cooking time: 10 minutes

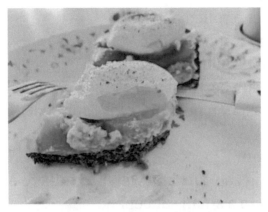

Avocado Toast with Eggs

Ingredients:
- 1 slice whole-wheat bread
- 1/4 avocado, mashed
- 1 egg, cooked to your liking
- Salt and pepper to taste

Preparation:
- Toast the bread.
- Spread the mashed avocado on the toast.
- Top with the cooked egg.
- Season with salt and pepper to taste. Enjoy!

Nutritional value (per serving):
- Calories: 250

- Protein: 12 grams
- Fat: 15 grams
- Carbohydrates: 20 grams
- Fibre: 5 grams

Cooking time: 10 minutes

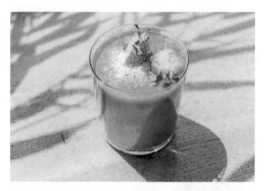

Smoothie with Protein Powder, Fruits, and Vegetables

Ingredients:
- 1 cup unsweetened almond milk
- 1 scoop protein powder
- 1/2 banana
- 1/2 cup berries
- 1/4 cup spinach

Preparation:
- Combine all ingredients in a blender and blend until smooth.Enjoy!

Nutritional value (per serving):
- Calories: 250
- Protein: 20 grams
- Fat: 10 grams
- Carbohydrates: 20 grams
- Fiber: 5 grams

Cooking time: 5 minutes

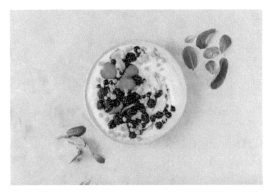

Overnight Oats with Yogurt, Fruits, and Nuts

Ingredients:
- 1/2 cup rolled oats
- 1/2 cup yogurt
- 1/4 cup milk of your choice
- 1/4 cup berries
- 1 tablespoon nuts or seeds

Preparation:
- Combine all ingredients in a jar or container.
- Stir to combine.
- Cover and refrigerate overnight.
- Enjoy in the morning!

Nutritional value (per serving):
- Calories: 250
- Protein: 10 grams
- Fat: 10 grams
- Carbohydrates: 30 grams
- Fibre: 5 grams

Cooking time: 5 minutes (plus overnight refrigeration)

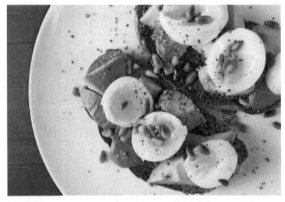

Hard-Boiled Eggs with Whole-Wheat Toast

Ingredients:
- 2 hard-boiled eggs
- 1 slice whole-wheat toast

Preparation:
- Peel and slice the hard-boiled eggs.
- Toast the bread.
- Top the toast with the sliced eggs.Enjoy!

Nutritional value (per serving):
- Calories: 200
- Protein: 12 grams
- Fat: 10 grams
- Carbohydrates: 20 grams

- Fiber: 5 grams

Cooking time: 15 minutes (plus time to hard-boil the eggs)

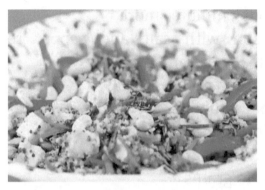

Tofu Scramble with Vegetables

Ingredients:
- 1/2 block tofu, crumbled
- 1/4 cup chopped onion
- 1/4 cup chopped bell pepper
- 1/4 cup chopped mushrooms
- 1/4 cup chopped spinach
- 1 tablespoon olive oil
- Salt and pepper to taste

Preparation:
- Heat the olive oil in a large skillet over medium heat.

- Add the onion, bell pepper, and mushrooms and cook until softened, about 5 minutes.
- Add the tofu and spinach and cook until the tofu is heated through, about 3 minutes more.
- Season with salt and pepper to taste.Serve immediately.

Nutritional value (per serving):
- Calories: 200
- Protein: 15 grams
- Fat: 10 grams
- Carbohydrates: 15 grams
- Fiber: 5 grams

Cooking time: 10 minutes

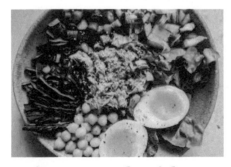

Quinoa Bowl with Avocado, Eggs, and Vegetables

Ingredients:
- 1/2 cup cooked quinoa
- 1/4 avocado, mashed
- 1 egg, cooked to your liking
- 1/4 cup chopped vegetables (tomatoes, cucumbers, onions, etc.)
- 1 tablespoon olive oil
- Salt and pepper to taste

Preparation:
- Combine the quinoa, avocado, egg, and vegetables in a bowl.
- Drizzle with olive oil and season with salt and pepper to taste.Enjoy!

Nutritional value (per serving):
- Calories: 300
- Protein: 15 grams
- Fat: 15 grams
- Carbohydrates: 25 grams
- Fiber: 5 grams

Cooking time: 10 minutes (plus time to cook the quinoa)

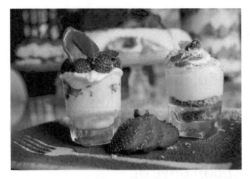

Chia Pudding with Berries and Nuts

Ingredients:
- 1/2 cup chia seeds
- 1 cup unsweetened almond milk
- 1/4 cup berries
- 1 tablespoon nuts or seeds

Preparation:
- Combine the chia seeds and almond milk in a jar or container.
- Stir to combine.
- Cover and refrigerate overnight.
- In the morning, top with berries and nuts.Enjoy!

Nutritional value (per serving):
- Calories: 250
- Protein: 10 grams

- Fat: 10 grams
- Carbohydrates: 30 grams
- Fibre: 5 grams

Cooking time: 5 minutes (plus overnight refrigeration)

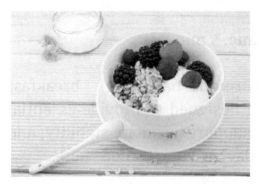

Yoghourt parfait with berries, nuts, and granola

Ingredients:
- 1 cup Greek yoghurt
- 1/4 cup berries
- 1/4 cup nuts or seeds
- 1/4 cup granola

Preparation:
- Layer the yoghurt, berries, nuts, and granola in a jar or glass.Enjoy!

Nutritional value (per serving):

- Calories: 300
- Protein: 20 grams
- Fat: 10 grams
- Carbohydrates: 30 grams
- Fibre: 5 grams

Cooking time: 5 minutes

These hormone-balancing breakfast recipes are designed to provide essential nutrients, support hormone stability, and start your day on a harmonious note.

By incorporating these recipes into your morning routine, you can take a proactive step toward managing the symptoms of menopause, nurturing emotional well-being, and embracing a holistic approach to this transformative phase of life.

CHAPTER 4

Satisfying and Nourishing Lunches

Lunch is the refuelling point in your day, providing the sustenance and energy needed to power through the afternoon.

During menopause, it's essential to choose meals that not only satisfy your hunger but also support your overall health and hormonal balance.

In this chapter, we will explore eight menopause-friendly lunch recipes, complete with ingredients, preparation methods, nutritional value, and cooking times.

These lunches are designed to keep you energised and feeling your best as you navigate the changes and challenges of menopause.

Nourishing Your Body at Noon

Lunch is an opportunity to replenish your energy and nourish your body with essential nutrients. As you navigate menopause, choosing the right foods can help stabilise hormone levels, improve mood, and support overall well-being.

A well-balanced midday meal can:

Provide sustained energy throughout the afternoon.

Stabilise blood sugar levels, reducing mood swings and irritability.

Deliver a variety of vitamins and minerals crucial for health.

Support hormonal balance and alleviate common menopausal symptoms.

By focusing on nutrient-dense and hormone-balancing foods, your lunch can be a cornerstone of your menopausal well-being.

Menopause-Friendly Lunch Recipes

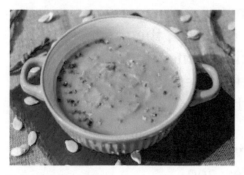

Lentil Soup

Ingredients:
- 1 cup lentils
- 2 cups vegetable broth
- 1 onion, chopped
- 2 carrots, chopped
- 2 celery stalks, chopped
- 1 teaspoon garlic powder
- 1/2 teaspoon dried thyme
- 1/4 teaspoon salt
- 1/4 teaspoon black pepper

Preparation:
- Rinse the lentils.

- Combine the lentils, vegetable broth, onion, carrots, celery, garlic powder, thyme, salt, and pepper in a large pot.
- Bring to a boil, then reduce heat to low and simmer for 20-30 minutes, or until the lentils are tender.
- Serve hot.

Nutritional value (per serving):
- Calories: 200
- Protein: 15 grams
- Fat: 5 grams
- Carbohydrates: 30 grams
- Fiber: 10 grams

Cooking time: 30 minutes

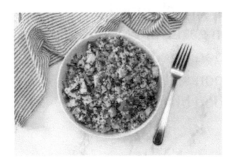

Quinoa Salad with Avocado, Tomatoes, and Cucumber

Ingredients:
- 1 cup cooked quinoa
- 1/2 avocado, diced
- 1/2 cup chopped tomatoes
- 1/2 cup chopped cucumber
- 1/4 cup chopped red onion
- 2 tablespoons olive oil
- 1 tablespoon lemon juice
- Salt and pepper to taste

Preparation:
- Combine the quinoa, avocado, tomatoes, cucumber, and red onion in a large bowl.
- Drizzle with olive oil and lemon juice.
- Season with salt and pepper to taste.
- Serve immediately.

Nutritional value (per serving):
- Calories: 300
- Protein: 10 grams
- Fat: 15 grams
- Carbohydrates: 30 grams
- Fiber: 10 grams

Cooking time: 10 minutes

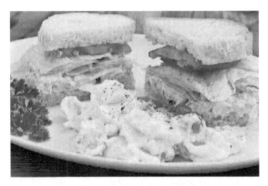

Tuna Salad Sandwich

Ingredients:
- 2 slices whole-wheat bread
- 1/4 cup canned tuna
- 1 tablespoon mayonnaise
- 1/4 cup chopped celery
- 1 tablespoon chopped red onion
- Salt and pepper to taste

Preparation:
- Mash the tuna in a bowl.
- Add the mayonnaise, celery, red onion, salt, and pepper.
- Mix well.
- Spread the tuna salad on the bread slices.

- Sandwich together and enjoy!

Nutritional value (per serving):
- Calories: 250
- Protein: 15 grams
- Fat: 10 grams
- Carbohydrates: 25 grams
- Fiber: 5 grams

Cooking time: 5 minutes

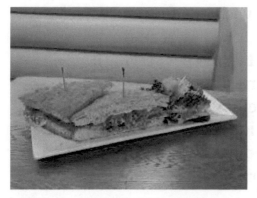

Salmon Salad Sandwich

Ingredients:
- 2 slices whole-wheat bread
- 1/4 cup canned salmon
- 1 tablespoon mayonnaise
- 1 tablespoon Dijon mustard

- 1/4 cup chopped celery
- 1 tablespoon chopped red onion
- Salt and pepper to taste

Preparation:
- Mash the salmon in a bowl.
- Add the mayonnaise, mustard, celery, red onion, salt, and pepper.
- Mix well.
- Spread the salmon salad on the bread slices.
- Sandwich together and enjoy!

Nutritional value (per serving):
- Calories: 300
- Protein: 15 grams
- Fat: 10 grams
- Carbohydrates: 30 grams
- Fiber: 5 grams

Cooking time: 5 minutes

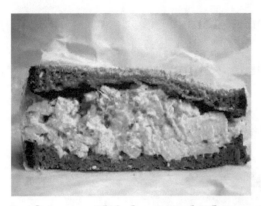

Leftover Chicken Salad Sandwich

Ingredients:
- 2 slices whole-wheat bread
- 1/2 cup leftover chicken salad
- Salt and pepper to taste

Preparation:
- Spread the leftover chicken salad on the bread slices.
- Season with salt and pepper to taste.
- Sandwich together and enjoy!

Nutritional value (per serving):
- Calories: 250
- Protein: 15 grams
- Fat: 10 grams
- Carbohydrates: 25 grams

- Fiber: 5 grams

Cooking time: 5 minutes

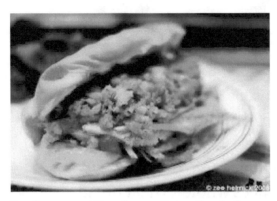

Leftover Turkey Sandwich

Ingredients:
- 2 slices whole-wheat bread
- 1/2 cup leftover turkey
- 1/4 cup lettuce
- 1/4 cup tomato slices
- 1 tablespoon mayonnaise or mustard (optional)

Preparation:
- Spread the mayonnaise or mustard on the bread slices (optional).

- Layer the turkey, lettuce, and tomato slices on the bread.
- Sandwich together and enjoy!

Nutritional value (per serving):
- Calories: 250
- Protein: 20 grams
- Fat: 5 grams
- Carbohydrates: 25 grams
- Fiber: 5 grams

Cooking time: 5 minutes

Leftover Lentil Soup

Ingredients:
- 1 cup leftover lentil soup
- 1 slice whole-wheat bread, toasted (optional)

Preparation:
- Heat up the leftover lentil soup.
- Serve with toasted bread (optional).

Nutritional value (per serving):
- Calories: 200

- Protein: 15 grams
- Fat: 5 grams
- Carbohydrates: 30 grams
- Fiber: 10 grams

Cooking time: 5 minutes

These satisfying and nourishing lunch recipes are carefully crafted to provide the essential nutrients needed to keep you energised and support your well-being during menopause.

By incorporating these recipes into your midday routine, you can make the most of your day, tackle menopausal challenges with vitality, and enjoy satisfying and nourishing meals that promote hormonal balance.

CHAPTER 5

Dinners to Soothe and Rejuvenate

Dinner is the closing act of your day, and it sets the stage for a restful night's sleep, which is crucial for hormonal balance during menopause.

In this chapter, we will explore ten hormone-balancing dinner recipes, complete with ingredients, preparation methods, nutritional value, and cooking times. These dinners are designed to soothe your body, rejuvenate your energy, and ensure a peaceful night's sleep.

A Hormone-Balancing Evening

As you approach evening, your focus should be on nurturing your body with foods that support hormonal balance and promote restfulness. A well-balanced dinner can:

Stabilise blood sugar levels, reducing night sweats and mood swings.

Provide essential nutrients to support hormonal health.

Offer a sense of satiety without overloading your digestive system.

Create a calming and comforting atmosphere for your evening routine.

By selecting hormone-balancing foods and recipes, you can turn your dinner into a nourishing ritual that contributes to a peaceful and restorative night.

Hormone-Balancing Dinner Recipes

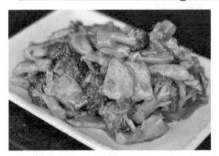

Chicken and Broccoli Stir-Fry

Ingredients:
- 1 pound boneless, skinless chicken breasts, cut into bite-sized pieces
- 1 tablespoon cornstarch
- 1 tablespoon olive oil
- 1/2 cup chopped onion
- 1 cup chopped broccoli florets
- 1/4 cup chopped red bell pepper
- 1/4 cup soy sauce
- 1 tablespoon rice vinegar
- 1 teaspoon sesame oil
- 1/4 teaspoon ground black pepper

Instructions:
- In a medium bowl, combine the chicken and cornstarch. Toss to coat.
- Heat the olive oil in a large skillet or wok over medium-high heat.
- Add the chicken and cook until browned on all sides.
- Add the onion, broccoli, and red bell pepper. Cook until the vegetables are tender.

- In a small bowl, whisk together the soy sauce, rice vinegar, sesame oil, and black pepper.
- Add the soy sauce mixture to the skillet and cook until the sauce is thickened.S
- erve immediately over rice or noodles.

Nutritional value (per serving):
- Calories: 250
- Protein: 30 grams
- Fat: 5 grams
- Carbohydrates: 20 grams
- Fiber: 5 grams

Cooking time: 20 minutes

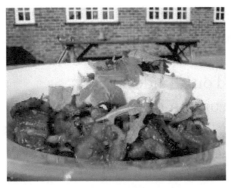

Salmon with Roasted Vegetables

Ingredients:

- 1 pound salmon fillet
- 1 tablespoon olive oil
- 1/2 teaspoon salt
- 1/4 teaspoon black pepper
- 1 cup broccoli florets
- 1 cup Brussels sprouts, halved
- 1/2 cup sweet potato, diced
- 1/4 teaspoon garlic powder
- 1/4 teaspoon onion powder

Instructions:

- Preheat oven to 400 degrees F (200 degrees C).
- Place the salmon fillet on a baking sheet lined with parchment paper.
- Drizzle with olive oil and season with salt and pepper.
- In a separate bowl, combine the broccoli, Brussels sprouts, sweet potato, garlic powder, and onion powder.
- Spread the vegetables around the salmon on the baking sheet.

- Bake for 20-25 minutes, or until the salmon is cooked through and the vegetables are tender.
- Serve immediately.

Nutritional value (per serving):
- Calories: 300
- Protein: 35 grams
- Fat: 10 grams
- Carbohydrates: 20 grams
- Fiber: 5 grams

Cooking time: 25 minutes

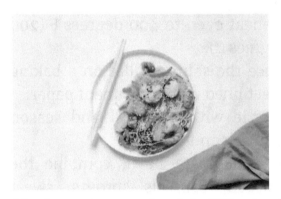

Shrimp Scampi with Whole-Wheat Pasta

Ingredients:
- 1 pound shrimp, peeled and deveined

- 1 tablespoon olive oil
- 1/4 cup chopped onion
- 2 cloves garlic, minced
- 1/4 cup dry white wine
- 1/4 cup lemon juice
- 1/4 cup chicken broth
- 1/4 teaspoon dried parsley
- 1/4 teaspoon dried thyme
- 1/4 teaspoon salt
- 1/4 teaspoon black pepper
- 8 ounces whole-wheat pasta

Instructions:
- Cook the pasta according to package directions.
- While the pasta is cooking, heat the olive oil in a large skillet or wok over medium-high heat.
- Add the shrimp and cook until pink and cooked through.
- Add the onion and garlic and cook until softened.
- Add the white wine, lemon juice, chicken broth, parsley, thyme, salt, and pepper. Bring to a boil, then reduce heat to low and simmer for 5 minutes.

- Drain the pasta and add it to the skillet with the shrimp and sauce. Toss to coat.
- Serve immediately.

Nutritional value (per serving):
- Calories: 350
- Protein: 35 grams
- Fat: 10 grams
- Carbohydrates: 30 grams
- Fiber: 5 grams

Cooking time: 20 minutes

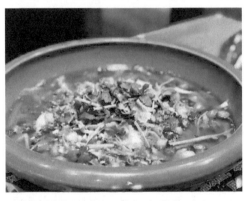

Lentil and Vegetable Soup

Ingredients:
- 1 cup lentils

- 2 cups vegetable broth
- 1 onion, chopped
- 2 carrots, chopped
- 2 celery stalks, chopped
- 1 teaspoon garlic powder
- 1/2 teaspoon dried thyme
- 1/4 teaspoon salt
- 1/4 teaspoon black pepper
- 1 (14.5 ounce) can diced tomatoes, undrained

Instructions:
- Rinse the lentils.
- In a large pot, combine the lentils, vegetable broth, onion, carrots, celery, garlic powder, thyme, salt, and pepper.
- Bring to a boil, then reduce heat to low and simmer for 20-30 minutes, or until the lentils are tender.
- Stir in the diced tomatoes and simmer for an additional 10 minutes.Serve hot.

Nutritional value (per serving):
- Calories: 200
- Protein: 15 grams

- Fat: 5 grams
- Carbohydrates: 30 grams
- Fiber: 10 grams

Cooking time: 30 minutes

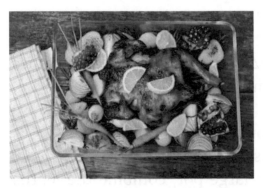

Chicken and Sweet Potato Curry

Ingredients:
- 1 pound boneless, skinless chicken breasts, cut into bite-sized pieces
- 1 tablespoon olive oil
- 1/2 cup chopped onion
- 2 cloves garlic, minced
- 1 tablespoon curry powder
- 1 teaspoon ground cumin
- 1/2 teaspoon ground turmeric
- 1/4 teaspoon salt
- 1/4 teaspoon black pepper

- 1 (14.5 ounce) can diced tomatoes, undrained
- 1 (15 ounce) can sweet potato puree
- 1/2 cup coconut milk

Instructions:
- Heat the olive oil in a large skillet or pot over medium heat.
- Add the chicken and cook until browned on all sides.
- Add the onion, garlic, curry powder, cumin, turmeric, salt, and pepper. Cook for 1 minute, stirring constantly.
- Stir in the diced tomatoes, sweet potato puree, and coconut milk. Bring to a boil, then reduce heat to low and simmer for 20 minutes, or until the chicken is cooked through and the sauce has thickened.
- Serve over rice or quinoa.

Nutritional value (per serving):
- Calories: 350
- Protein: 30 grams
- Fat: 10 grams
- Carbohydrates: 30 grams

- Fiber: 5 grams
- Cooking time: 30 minutes

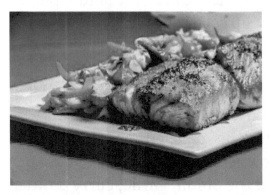

Salmon with Roasted Vegetables and Quinoa

Ingredients:
- 1 pound salmon fillet
- 1 tablespoon olive oil
- 1/2 teaspoon salt
- 1/4 teaspoon black pepper
- 1 (16 ounce) bag frozen mixed vegetables, thawed
- 1 cup cooked quinoa

Instructions:
- Preheat oven to 400 degrees F (200 degrees C).

- Place the salmon fillet on a baking sheet lined with parchment paper.
- Drizzle with olive oil and season with salt and pepper.
- Spread the mixed vegetables around the salmon on the baking sheet.
- Bake for 20-25 minutes, or until the salmon is cooked through and the vegetables are tender.
- Serve immediately over quinoa.

Nutritional value (per serving):
- Calories: 400
- Protein: 35 grams
- Fat: 15 grams
- Carbohydrates: 35 grams
- Fiber: 5 grams

Cooking time: 25 minutes

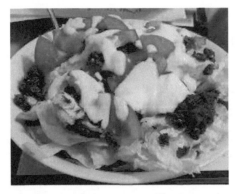

Vegetarian Lentil Taco Bowl

Ingredients:
- 1 cup cooked lentils
- 1/2 cup chopped lettuce
- 1/4 cup chopped tomato
- 1/4 cup chopped avocado
- 1/4 cup chopped red onion
- 1 tablespoon taco seasoning
- 1 tablespoon salsa
- 1/4 cup tortilla chips

Instructions:
- In a bowl, combine the lentils, lettuce, tomato, avocado, red onion, taco seasoning, and salsa.
- Serve over tortilla chips.

Nutritional value (per serving):
- Calories: 300
- Protein: 15 grams
- Fat: 10 grams
- Carbohydrates: 35 grams
- Fiber: 5 grams

Cooking time: 10 minutes

Tofu Stir-Fry with Brown Rice

Ingredients:
- 1 block tofu, crumbled
- 1 tablespoon olive oil
- 1/2 cup chopped onion
- 1/2 cup chopped bell pepper
- 1/2 cup chopped mushrooms
- 1/4 cup soy sauce
- 1 tablespoon rice vinegar
- 1 teaspoon sesame oil
- 1/4 teaspoon black pepper
- 1 cup cooked brown rice

Instructions:
- Heat the olive oil in a large skillet or wok over medium-high heat.

- Add the tofu and cook until browned on all sides.
- Add the onion, bell pepper, and mushrooms and cook until softened.
- Add the soy sauce, rice vinegar, sesame oil, and black pepper. Stir to combine.
- Serve over brown rice.

Nutritional value (per serving):
- Calories: 350
- Protein: 25 grams
- Fat: 10 grams
- Carbohydrates: 40 grams
- Fiber: 5 grams

Cooking time: 20 minutes

By incorporating these recipes into your midday routine, you can make the most of your day, tackle menopausal challenges with vitality, and enjoy satisfying and nourishing meals that promote hormonal balance.

CHAPTER 6

Revitalising Smoothies and Snacks

In the midst of a busy day, snacking can be a lifesaver, providing much-needed energy and nutrition to fuel your activities.

This chapter focuses on seven nutrient-packed smoothie and snack recipes, each designed to give you a revitalising boost.

We'll explore the ingredients, preparation methods, nutritional value, and cooking times to ensure that your snacks are not only delicious but also contribute to hormonal balance and well-being during menopause.

Energising Snacking During Menopause

Snacks play a crucial role in maintaining energy levels and preventing dips that can lead to mood swings and irritability. Choosing nutrient-dense options can make all the difference during menopause.

By incorporating hormone-balancing foods into your snacks, you can enjoy quick and healthy bites that revitalise and nourish your body.

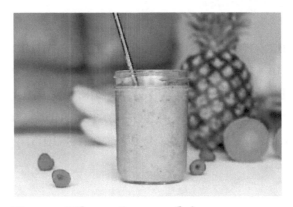

Berry Blast Smoothie

Ingredients:
- 1 cup of mixed berries (strawberries, blueberries, raspberries)
- 1 banana1 tablespoon of flaxseeds
- 1 cup of Greek yoghurt
- 1 cup of almond milk

Preparation:
- Blend all ingredients until smooth.

Nutritional Value:
- Calories: 250
- Protein: 12g
- Fiber: 8g

Cooking Time:5 minutes

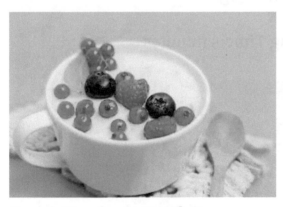

Greek Yoghurt Parfait

Ingredients:
- 1 cup of Greek yogurt
- 1/2 cup of granola
- 1/2 cup of mixed berries (strawberries, blueberries)
- 1 tablespoon of honey

Preparation:
- Layer yogurt, granola, and berries in a glass or bowl.
- Drizzle with honey.

Nutritional Value:
- Calories: 320
- Protein: 20g
- Fiber: 6g

Cooking Time: 5 minutes

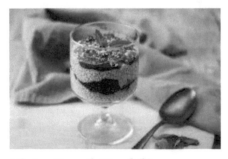

Chia Seed Pudding

Ingredients:
- 3 tablespoons of chia seeds
- 1 cup of almond milk
- 1/2 teaspoon of vanilla extract
- 1/2 cup of sliced kiwi and strawberries
- 1 tablespoon of honey

Preparation:
- Mix chia seeds, almond milk, and vanilla extract in a jar. Refrigerate overnight.
- In the morning, top with sliced fruits and drizzle with honey.

Nutritional Value:
- Calories: 280
- Protein: 7g
- Fiber: 15g

Cooking Time: 5 minutes (plus overnight refrigeration)

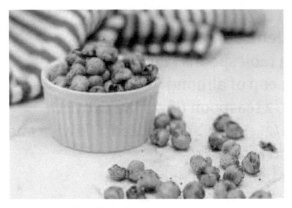

Roasted Chickpeas

Ingredients:
- 1 can of chickpeas, drained and rinsed
- 1 tablespoon of olive oil
- 1 teaspoon of paprika and cumin
- Salt and pepper to taste

Preparation:
- Toss chickpeas in olive oil, paprika, cumin, salt, and pepper.
- Roast in the oven until crispy.

Nutritional Value:
- Calories: 160
- Protein: 5g
- Fiber: 5g

Cooking Time: 30 minutes

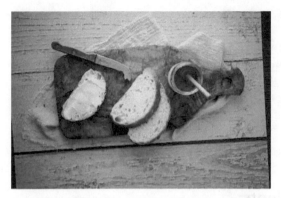

Apple Slices with Almond Butter

Ingredients:
- 1 apple, sliced
- 2 tablespoons of almond butter

Preparation:
- Dip apple slices in almond butter.

Nutritional Value:
- Calories: 220
- Protein: 4g
- Fiber: 5g

Cooking Time: 5 minutes

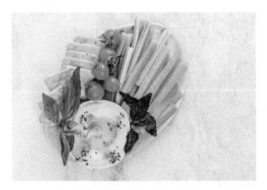

Veggie Sticks with Hummus

Ingredients:
- 1 cup of carrot and cucumber sticks
- 1/4 cup of hummus

Preparation:
- Dip veggie sticks in hummus.

Nutritional Value:
- Calories: 140
- Protein: 3g
- Fiber: 5g

Cooking Time: 5 minutes

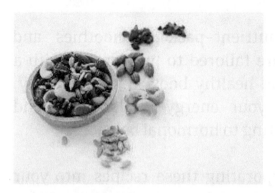

Trail Mix with Nuts and Dried Fruit

Ingredients:
- 1/4 cup of mixed nuts (almonds, walnuts, cashews)
- 1/4 cup of dried fruit (apricots, cranberries, raisins)
- 1/4 cup of dark chocolate chips

Preparation:
- Mix nuts, dried fruit, and chocolate chips in a bowl.

Nutritional Value:
- Calories: 280
- Protein: 6g
- Fiber: 4g

Cooking Time: 5 minutes

These nutrient-packed smoothies and snacks are tailored to provide you with a quick and healthy boost during the day, keeping your energy levels stable and contributing to hormonal balance.

By incorporating these recipes into your snacking routine, you can enjoy revitalising bites that support your well-being during menopause.

CHAPTER 7

Satisfying Your Sweet Tooth Mindfully

Satisfying your sweet tooth doesn't have to be a guilty pleasure, especially during menopause. In this chapter, we'll explore five delicious dessert recipes tailored for menopausal women.

These desserts not only delight your taste buds but also contribute to hormonal balance and overall well-being.

We'll provide details on the ingredients, preparation methods, nutritional value, and cooking times to ensure that you can enjoy these treats mindfully.

Indulging in Healthy Desserts

During menopause, the desire for sweet treats may intensify, but it's essential to indulge in a way that aligns with your health goals.

Healthy desserts can be both satisfying and supportive of hormonal balance. A well-balanced dessert can:

Provide the sweetness you crave without the drawbacks of excessive sugar.

Deliver essential nutrients that benefit your health.

Keep you satisfied and reduce the risk of overindulgence.

By selecting hormone-balancing ingredients and recipes, you can enjoy dessert without compromising your well-being.

Delicious Dessert Recipes for Menopausal Women

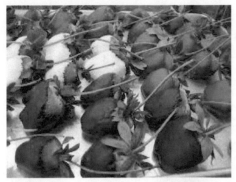

Dark Chocolate-Dipped Strawberries

Ingredients:
- 1 cup of fresh strawberries
- 3 oz of dark chocolate (70% cocoa or higher)

Preparation:
- Melt the dark chocolate in a microwave or on a stovetop.
- Dip each strawberry in the melted chocolate and let them cool on parchment paper.

Nutritional Value:
- Calories: 150
- Protein: 2g
- Fiber: 3g

Cooking Time:15 minutes

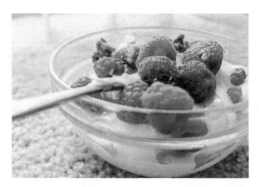

Greek Yogurt with Honey and Berries

Ingredients:
- 1 cup of Greek yogurt
- 1 tablespoon of honey
- 1/2 cup of mixed berries (blueberries, raspberries)

Preparation:
- Top Greek yogurt with honey and mixed berries.

Nutritional Value:
- Calories: 200
- Protein: 14g

- Fiber: 3g

Cooking Time:5 minutes

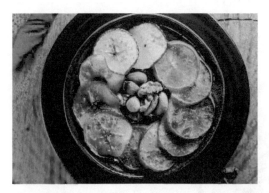

Baked Apples with Cinnamon and Walnuts

Ingredients:
- 2 apples, cored and halved
- 1 teaspoon of cinnamon
- 2 tablespoons of chopped walnuts
- 1 tablespoon of honey

Preparation:
- Sprinkle apples with cinnamon and bake until tender.
- Top with chopped walnuts and drizzle with honey.

Nutritional Value:
- Calories: 250
- Protein: 3g
- Fiber: 6g

Cooking Time: 30 minutes

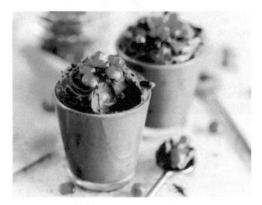

Chia Seed Chocolate Pudding

Ingredients:
- 3 tablespoons of chia seeds
- 1 cup of almond milk
- 2 tablespoons of unsweetened cocoa powder
- 1/2 teaspoon of vanilla extract
- 1 tablespoon of maple syrup

Preparation:
- Mix chia seeds, almond milk, cocoa powder, vanilla extract, and maple syrup in a jar. Refrigerate until it thickens.

Nutritional Value:
- Calories: 220
- Protein: 6g
- Fiber: 12g

Cooking Time:5 minutes (plus refrigeration)

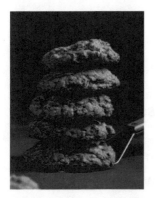

Banana and Almond Oat Cookies

Ingredients:
- 2 ripe bananas, mashed
- 1 cup of rolled oats
- 1/4 cup of almond butter

- 1/4 cup of dark chocolate chips
- 1/2 teaspoon of vanilla extract

Preparation:
- Mix mashed bananas, oats, almond butter, dark chocolate chips, and vanilla extract in a bowl.
- Drop spoonfuls of the mixture onto a baking sheet and bake until golden.

Nutritional Value:
- Calories: 180
- Protein: 4g
- Fibre: 4g

Cooking Time: 20 minutes

These delicious dessert recipes are thoughtfully designed to satisfy your sweet tooth while promoting hormonal balance and overall well-being during menopause.

By incorporating these recipes into your dessert options, you can enjoy delightful treats mindfully and indulge in a way that supports your health.

CHAPTER 8

The Menopause Reset Meal Plans

In this chapter, we provide you with thoughtfully designed meal plans tailored to menopause. These plans include balanced combinations of nutrient-dense foods, recipes, and portion sizes to support hormonal balance and overall well-being during this life stage.

The meal plans offer a practical guide to help you make healthy choices, manage symptoms, and enjoy satisfying, menopause-friendly meals.

14-Day Hormone-Balancing Meal Plan for Menopause

Day 1

Breakfast: Greek yoghurt with mixed berries and honey.Whole grain toast with almond butter.

Lunch: Grilled chicken salad with mixed greens, cherry tomatoes, and balsamic vinaigrette.Quinoa side dish.

Dinner: Baked salmon with asparagus.Steamed broccoli with a sprinkle of Parmesan cheese.

Snack: A small handful of nuts and dried apricots.

Day 2

Breakfast: Spinach and feta omelet.Whole grain toast.

Lunch: Lentil and spinach soup.Whole grain crackers.

Dinner: Quinoa-stuffed bell peppers.Side of mixed greens.

Snack: Sliced cucumbers with hummus.

Day 3

Breakfast: Chia seed pudding with fresh mango and a drizzle of honey.

Lunch: Veggie and quinoa stuffed peppers.Side salad with vinaigrette.

Dinner: Baked sweet potato with black bean salsa.Steamed green beans.

Snack: A piece of dark chocolate.

Day 4

Breakfast: Mixed berry smoothie with spinach, chia seeds, and Greek yogurt.

Lunch: Grilled chicken and vegetable stir-fry.Brown rice.

Dinner: Tofu and vegetable stir-fry.Steamed broccoli.

Snack: Greek yogurt with sliced strawberries.

Day 5

Breakfast: Scrambled eggs with sautéed spinach and a sprinkle of feta cheese.

Lunch: Quinoa and black bean salad with corn and red pepper.

Dinner: Shrimp and broccoli stir-fry.Brown rice.

Snack: Sliced apple with almond butter.

Day 6

Breakfast: Baked apple with cinnamon and walnuts.A dollop of Greek yogurt.

Lunch: Caprese salad with grilled chicken.

Dinner: Grilled salmon with lemon and dill.Roasted asparagus.

Snack: Trail mix with mixed nuts and dried fruit.

Day 7

Breakfast: Banana and almond oat cookies.A glass of almond milk.

Lunch: Spinach and strawberry salad with grilled chicken and balsamic dressing.

Dinner: Balsamic glazed chicken with roasted vegetables.

Snack: A small piece of dark chocolate.

Day 8-14

Feel free to repeat the meals from days 1-7 for days 8-14, making sure to include a variety of nutrient-dense and hormone-balancing foods in your daily meals. Adapt portion sizes and ingredients to your preferences and dietary needs.

20 healthy Grocery Shopping list to Success

Fresh Fruits: Apples, bananas, berries, oranges, and any of your favourites. Fruits are rich in vitamins, fibre, and antioxidants.

Fresh Vegetables: Leafy greens, broccoli, carrots, bell peppers, and other colorful vegetables. They provide essential nutrients and fibre.

Lean Proteins: Skinless poultry, lean cuts of beef, tofu, or plant-based protein sources like beans and lentils. Protein is vital for muscle health and feeling full.

Fatty Fish: Salmon, sardines, or mackerel. These are rich in omega-3 fatty acids, which support heart and brain health.

Whole Grains: Brown rice, quinoa, whole wheat pasta, and oats. Whole grains provide sustained energy and fibre.

Dairy or Dairy Alternatives: Low-fat or non-fat yogurt, milk, or dairy-free alternatives like almond or soy milk.

Eggs: A versatile source of protein and essential nutrients.

Nuts and Seeds: Almonds, walnuts, chia seeds, and flaxseeds. These are rich in healthy fats and fiber.

Healthy Cooking Oils: Olive oil, avocado oil, or coconut oil. These are better alternatives to heavily processed oils.

Herbs and Spices: Cinnamon, turmeric, basil, and others. These add flavour and have potential health benefits.

Lean Deli Meats: Turkey or chicken breast, sliced thinly for sandwiches or salads.

Whole-Grain Bread or Wraps: Choose options with minimal additives and high fiber content.

Low-Fat Cheese: A source of calcium and protein.

Greek Yogurt: High in protein and probiotics, which promote gut health.

Canned Beans and Tomatoes: Great for adding to soups, stews, or salads.

Frozen Fruits and Vegetables: These are convenient and often as nutritious as fresh.

Nut Butter: Natural peanut butter or almond butter with minimal added sugars.

Hydration Options: Water, herbal tea, or unsweetened beverages. Staying hydrated is crucial.

Snack Items: Hummus, whole-grain crackers, and fresh popcorn for healthier snacking.

Dark Chocolate: In moderation, it can satisfy your sweet tooth while providing antioxidants.

Tips for a Successful Grocery Shopping Trip:

Plan your meals for the week in advance to ensure you have all the necessary ingredients.

Stick to your list to avoid impulse purchases.

Shop the perimeter of the store, where fresh produce, meats, and dairy are usually located, to focus on whole foods.

Check food labels for added sugars, trans fats, and artificial additives.

Buy in bulk for non-perishable items like grains and canned goods to save money.

Creating a healthy grocery shopping list is a proactive step towards improving your overall nutrition and well-being. Remember to choose a variety of foods to ensure a balanced and diverse diet.

CHAPTER 9

Staying Mentally Fit and Emotionally Balanced

Menopause is a significant life transition that every woman will experience, and it brings about a multitude of physical changes.

However, what often takes a back seat in the discussions about menopause is its profound impact on mental and emotional well-being.

The hormonal fluctuations that characterise this phase can create a rollercoaster of emotions and cognitive changes, but with the right strategies, it's possible to stay mentally fit and emotionally balanced.

Understanding the Impact of Menopause on Mental Health

Menopause is more than just the cessation of menstrual periods; it marks a fundamental shift in hormonal balance. The most notable change is the decline in estrogen, a hormone that plays a crucial role in brain function.

As oestrogen levels drop, many women experience a range of cognitive and emotional changes. Some of the common symptoms include:

Mood Swings: Fluctuations in estrogen can lead to mood swings, irritability, and emotional volatility. You might find yourself feeling anxious, easily frustrated, or downcast.

Memory and Concentration Issues: Many women report difficulties with memory, focus, and cognitive function during menopause. Forgetfulness and mental fog become frequent companions.

Sleep Disturbances: Hormonal changes can disrupt sleep patterns, leading to insomnia or poor-quality sleep. Sleep is essential for cognitive function and emotional stability.

Anxiety and Depression: The hormonal shifts can trigger or exacerbate anxiety and depression. The increased emotional sensitivity can make these conditions more challenging to manage.

Stress and Coping Mechanisms: The pressures of daily life can feel more overwhelming during menopause. Coping mechanisms that worked in the past might become less effective.

Strategies for Coping and Thriving

While these mental and emotional challenges are part of the menopausal journey, they are not insurmountable.

With the right strategies and support, you can navigate this phase with resilience and grace. Here are some practical approaches to help you stay mentally fit and emotionally balanced:

<u>**Maintain a Healthy Lifestyle**</u>:

Diet: A balanced diet rich in fruits, vegetables, whole grains, lean proteins, and healthy fats can support cognitive function and mood stability.

Exercise: Regular physical activity can reduce stress, improve mood, and enhance cognitive function. Aim for at least 150 minutes of moderate-intensity exercise per week.

Sleep: Prioritise good sleep hygiene by creating a dark, cool, and quiet sleep environment. Establish a regular sleep schedule and avoid stimulating activities before bedtime.

Hormone Replacement Therapy (HRT):

Discuss the potential benefits and risks of HRT with your healthcare provider. HRT can help alleviate some menopausal symptoms and support emotional well-being.

Cognitive Behavioral Therapy (CBT):

CBT is an evidence-based therapy that can help you manage anxiety, depression, and stress.

It focuses on changing negative thought patterns and developing effective coping strategies.

Mindfulness and Meditation:

Mindfulness practices, such as meditation and deep breathing exercises, can reduce stress, improve emotional regulation, and enhance overall well-being.

Social Support:

Connect with friends and loved ones. Sharing your experiences and feelings can be therapeutic. Strong social connections are linked to better mental health.

Cognitive Training:

Engage in activities that challenge your brain, such as puzzles, crosswords, or learning a new skill.

Cognitive training can help combat memory and cognitive issues.

Herbal and Natural Remedies:

Some women find relief from symptoms using herbal supplements like black cohosh, evening primrose oil, or St. John's Wort.

Consult with a healthcare provider before using any natural remedies.

Stress Management:

Explore stress-reduction techniques like yoga, tai chi, or progressive muscle relaxation. These practices can help you better cope with life's pressures.

Emotional Self-Care:

Prioritize self-care activities that bring you joy and relaxation. It might be reading, gardening, painting, or simply taking a soothing bath.

Professional Help:

If you find that your mental and emotional well-being is significantly impacted, don't hesitate to seek professional help. A therapist or counsellor can provide valuable support and guidance.

Mental and emotional wellness during menopause is about self-compassion, adaptability, and resilience.

The journey may have its challenges, but it also offers an opportunity for personal growth and self-discovery. By implementing these strategies and seeking support when needed, you can embrace this phase of life with a sense of empowerment and emotional equilibrium.

CONCLUSION

The Menopause Reset Diet isn't just a diet; it's a path to a healthier, happier menopausal journey.

We've explored the profound impact of nutrition on your physical and mental well-being during this life stage, and armed with this knowledge, you are now empowered to make choices that can transform the way you experience menopause.

Throughout this journey, we've discovered that the right foods can alleviate symptoms, support hormonal balance, and promote overall health.

You've learned how to create hormone-balancing meals, satisfy your cravings with healthy options, and nourish your body with nutrient-rich foods.

By incorporating hormone-balancing ingredients into your daily meals, you've taken a proactive step toward enhancing your overall well-being.

Menopause is a profound transition, a passage to the next chapter of your life, and you have the power to embrace it with grace and vitality.

By adopting and adapting to the Menopause Reset Diet, you're not just making dietary changes; you're making a commitment to yourself.

You're choosing to prioritise your health, to cherish the journey, and to celebrate the strength and resilience that define this phase of life.

In the words of Maya Angelou, "We all should know that diversity makes for a rich tapestry, and we must understand that all the threads of the tapestry are equal in value no matter their colour."

Menopause is a thread in the rich tapestry of your life, and with the Menopause Reset Diet, you have the means to weave it with vibrancy, vitality, and a profound sense of well-being.

So, let this journey be a celebration of your health, a testimony to your adaptability, and a testament to the power of the choices you make.

As you continue forward, know that you are not alone. Countless women are on this journey with you, all striving for health, happiness, and empowerment. The Menopause Reset Diet is your guiding light, illuminating the path to a brighter, more vibrant future.

Embrace the Menopause Reset Diet, nourish your body and soul, and embark on this new phase of life with strength, resilience, and boundless optimism. Your journey is just beginning, and the best is yet to come.

MY WEEKLY
MEAL JOURNAL

Start Date: _____

End Date: _____

MONDAY	BREAKFAST	
	LUNCH	
	DINNER	
TUESDAY	BREAKFAST	
	LUNCH	
	DINNER	
WEDNESDAY	BREAKFAST	
	LUNCH	
	DINNER	
THURSDAY	BREAKFAST	
	LUNCH	
	DINNER	
FRIDAY	BREAKFAST	
	LUNCH	
	DINNER	
SATURDAY	BREAKFAST	
	LUNCH	
	DINNER	
SUNDAY	BREAKFAST	
	LUNCH	
	DINNER	

GROCERY LIST

SNACKS

MY WEEKLY
MEAL JOURNAL

Start Date:_____

End Date:_____

MONDAY	BREAKFAST	
	LUNCH	
	DINNER	
TUESDAY	BREAKFAST	
	LUNCH	
	DINNER	
WEDNESDAY	BREAKFAST	
	LUNCH	
	DINNER	
THURSDAY	BREAKFAST	
	LUNCH	
	DINNER	
FRIDAY	BREAKFAST	
	LUNCH	
	DINNER	
SATURDAY	BREAKFAST	
	LUNCH	
	DINNER	
SUNDAY	BREAKFAST	
	LUNCH	
	DINNER	

GROCERY LIST

SNACKS

MY WEEKLY
MEAL JOURNAL

Start Date:_____

End Date:_____

MONDAY	BREAKFAST	
	LUNCH	
	DINNER	
TUESDAY	BREAKFAST	
	LUNCH	
	DINNER	
WEDNESDAY	BREAKFAST	
	LUNCH	
	DINNER	
THURSDAY	BREAKFAST	
	LUNCH	
	DINNER	
FRIDAY	BREAKFAST	
	LUNCH	
	DINNER	
SATURDAY	BREAKFAST	
	LUNCH	
	DINNER	
SUNDAY	BREAKFAST	
	LUNCH	
	DINNER	

GROCERY LIST

SNACKS

MY WEEKLY
MEAL JOURNAL

Start Date: _____

End Date: _____

MONDAY	BREAKFAST	
	LUNCH	
	DINNER	
TUESDAY	BREAKFAST	
	LUNCH	
	DINNER	
WEDNESDAY	BREAKFAST	
	LUNCH	
	DINNER	
THURSDAY	BREAKFAST	
	LUNCH	
	DINNER	
FRIDAY	BREAKFAST	
	LUNCH	
	DINNER	
SATURDAY	BREAKFAST	
	LUNCH	
	DINNER	
SUNDAY	BREAKFAST	
	LUNCH	
	DINNER	

GROCERY LIST

SNACKS

Made in United States
Troutdale, OR
05/17/2024

19907592R00070